How I Managed a Cure
for
Asthma
and other
Medical Problems

How I Managed a Cure for
Asthma and other Medical Problems
Copyright © 2016 E. S. Amons

Contents

Forward

I'm not writing a long, drawn out book just to increase the size of the book and have you read what I'll call 'fill in nothing words'. I'm flatly going to tell you what I went through with my son along with some medical issues about me and how cures to medical problems were found. I am also not going to mention the daily struggles and agony but I'm sure you will know that it was there.

I am not a medical person. I am just a baby boomer mom who fought like heck to get my son well with his daunting medical problems and saw success. I shocked a few doctors along the way.

My son was born in November 1966, gosh at fifty years ago as I write this book. About forty years ago was when all the medical problems were known and the cure began. The length of time without reoccurrences proves he was cured.

Thru the years I've told people of the varied medical problems he had and how I found a cure. Many have said, "You should write a book" from the beginning of the problems." Here it is.

Chapter One – The First Five Years

My son was born with a normal delivery, so I thought. The doctor had figured that I was two days overdue and he wanted to go on vacation so he called me personally and said he was going to put me in the hospital to induce labor. I got to the hospital a couple of days later as arranged and was scared to death as it was my first baby. There was no such thing then as classes to prepare the mother.

They got me to the labor area and the nurses kept feeding me little white pills, then more and further more. Finally labor set in. The 'water' had not broken when they wheeled me into delivery. They used gas on me so I remember nothing past that point. The birth was within six hours after they began the little white pills.

When I saw my baby I was worried as the entire one side of his face was completely indented and the sides of his head at the temple area were very red and somewhat indented. While still in the hospital when I saw the doctor, I questioned him about the face being indented and the red indents on the sides of his head. I was told that the face indent was because the baby had been against my spine and that caused the face indent. I was assured it would be normal in a week or so. Concerning the red and indents on the sides of his head, I was told that they had to use forceps and that the doctor had to pull hard to get the baby out. I didn't know what to say but I didn't like it one bit. I kept thinking and still do that he was not ready to be born.

We were kept in the hospital three days, the normal time frame back then and I was sent home with instructions for feedings. The indents on his head were all gone between two and three weeks later, not a week as was stated. They did not want the moms to 'breast feed' back then and I was given instructions for formula, plus pills to dry up my natural milk when we left the hospital. Along with doing sterilized bottles as was done back then, that first month was a nightmare and I was in a panic. He couldn't keep the formula down at all. It wasn't that he just spit up, it was a good three to four foot 'throw' when he would up-chuck his milk at every feeding. Under the instructions of the pediatrician we tried formula after formula before the right one was found and he could finally keep his feedings down. I don't remember all the different names of infant milk products he was put on other than one in the maze was Isomil.

It soon became time to introduce other things to his feedings besides baby cereal and his special milk and that didn't go to well at all. I remember I had to mix just a little of the baby food with his special milk for him to keep it down. I talked to the pediatrician about him having possible stomach problems and I was ignored. As it became time for him to eat warmed up straight food from the baby food jars that were heated in a pan of water, one food that would bring on the long range, heavy up-chuck was green beans but there were other foods that did that to him also. Green beans brought on the really heavy up-chucking.

All of his checkups at the pediatrician office went well. I was told that he was doing fine and that he was in the upper classification with however they gauged the development with children.

My son seemed to be really smart and advancing rapidly – until he began to walk. I noticed soon after he began to walk, totally walk, that he seemed to be declining with abilities, almost mentally for the lack of a better explanation. He didn't seem to be doing the advancement with what he could do and seemed to decline, move a little backwards in my opinion. When saying something about it to my mother-in-law a couple of times, she would say that he was fine and I was seeing things not there. My mother was deceased so she could not be consulted.

The second and third years of my sons life went along fairly normal except he definitely had a mind of his own. There were still foods he absolutely could not eat without doing his then famous 'up-chuck'. There was a day during his third year when we went on a camping trip when one of his eyes swelling up gigantically. We packed up and went home. I can only assume he touched a weed and then his eye. The doctor only said 'Use ice'.

By the time my son reached age four we had a personality problem to deal with. He was like the wild boy from the unknown dimension. He would not follow any instruction. He always wanted to move around as if not being able to sit still and he always seemed to have a cold.

Right after his third birthday, the Christmas of 1969 his grandparents got him a little metal red fire engine that he could sit and ride around in. He wanted nothing to do with it. We put him in it and he hung his head down hiding it behind his arm and acted like he wanted to cry. When asked a question while he was sitting there, he refused to talk. It was as if the toy put him into a trance. He was finally taken out of it and went to the other side of the room acting very sad. He hated that fire engine and never played with it. We don't know why and I cannot explain it other than it may have been a past life thing, if there is reincarnation.

An odd thing went on during his fourth and fifth years. He had poison ivy, so it was said, on one elbow. For two years he had to wear a bandage wrapped around that part of his arm along with special salve medication from the doctor. Finally after two years, one day it cleared up.

Chapter Two – The Sixth thru Tenth Year

By the sixth year the never ending runny nose was more than an inconvenience. Constantly he was at the family doctor and given various medications that did no good at all. Very often they would dish out antibiotic prescriptions for him. Three years later, in his ninth year, an elder family member said that she knew of a boy who was like that and it was allergies. I found out who the doctor was and he was a pediatric allergist. I made an appointment for testing and had to wait about a month to get in. The nose on my son was beyond raw. With that doctor my son was tested with a series of 'scratch tests'. It seems there were at least two different dates for two different types of scratch tests. As I remember it, they would do the test, then send you home and the next day or so you went back to have the results (the inflammation) read. I remember my son was in misery with the tests as they itched and stung badly. The end result was finally given to me. Their words were "He is the worst for allergies we have ever seen". He was put on weekly allergy shots which had to be special made just for him so meanwhile he was given some medication to ease up the stinging from the testing. I was warned that he would probably be worse for at least a month or so when the shots started and they gave me little white pills to give him if he had a bad allergy or asthma attack. I soon found out what 'attack' they were talking about. Right after the shots began he started having allergy problems where his throat would close up so badly that when he talked he sounded like he had a deep voice along with laryngitis. He had been having breathing problems and now they were worse too. I kept a supply of those little pills for years and made sure the school nurse had some too. As time moved forward every Wednesday evening we would make the drive for his weekly allergy shot and every year we would do retesting.

While in his first years of school it became apparent that there was a problem with his learning. He was learning absolutely nothing. His days were him causing upheavals in class, drawing, and anything except learning. The school called me in for meetings and I agreed for testing to try to figure out what his learning problems were. The end result after a lot of days and spent gasoline was that he had learning disabilities and soon after he was diagnosed as having dyslexia. That involved him actually being put into the 'retarded class', private tutors, counseling and a full year of him sitting in school doing nothing except drawing and coloring. I was beyond upset as we were in one of the best school systems. I was totally lost with what to do.

As if that wasn't enough, he also had a leg that stopped growing. Now we were dealing with an orthopedic surgeon on top of the allergy and school problems. The orthopedic surgeon did a battery of x-rays and put him in a special shoe that had a big clunky lift on the bottom of the shoe for the shorter leg. It was not a cheap thing to get and it had to be replaced about every six months or sooner per his growth. My son hated the shoes as they were solid black, ugly and was not anything like the other kids wore. I had to force him to wear them which gave me no brownie points with him.

The orthopedic surgeon said that when my son reached age fifteen or sixteen, depending on the growth, he wanted to stop the growth in the longer leg. That would involve a surgery to go into the growth nodes of his knee on the longer leg and destroy those growth nodes which would give the shorter leg time to grow.

My son also developed bowel problems. It was unbelievable what came out of him. There was no way it could be flushed down the toilet with the length and width. We had tried once too often to flush it and had a heck of a mess to clean up. It had to be scooped out and put in a bag for which my son was shown what to do. That is just the way it was and no doctor could offer any help. There was no magic remedy. Thinking back now, we should have had a bucket with a plastic bag in it set up for him.

The tally at the end of year ten that I was dealing with was the weekly allergy shots, the retesting for needed allergy shot changes, the home medications for bad asthma and allergy attacks, the weekly and at times bi-weekly tutors, the school things I was to be working with him at home on, summer school at a local college where the students used him as someone to learn about dyslexia with as they supposedly helped him learn, a stunted leg along with an upcoming surgery and special shoes, and with the over loaded toilet problem plus he had a very bad stuttering problem and was in speech therapy.

With everything we were dealing with we had reached a point, even though we had good medical insurance, that the cost to us was very extensive. I managed to get help thru the Ohio Crippled Childrens Fund that existed back then.

Chapter Three – The Eleventh thru Fifteenth Year

Meanwhile during all of the problems I was dealing with concerning my son, I had an excessive amount of my own medical problems. I was dealing with things the family doctor could not put a name too and really they didn't search for it. They had me drugged up on their so called 'magic pills' that made me feel worse and sent me to a psychiatrist as time moved on. It ended up that the psychiatrists were telling me their problems and I quit going as it was a waste of time when they told me they could find nothing wrong with me. Meanwhile, I knew I was in bad shape, but exactly what and why were mysteries.

I asked the family doctor if I could possibly have cysts on my spine somewhere causing any of my neurological strangeness as I had a lot of ganglion cysts removed in the past. Again without any testing I was told no. At that point I bought my own copy of Gray's Anatomy and hit the library to start reading. It took a year but I think I read every medical book in the library that had any reference to neurological problems and anything connected to what my son had wrong with him. My conclusion was that I and my son had something wrong neurologically with us but I couldn't make the connection of what it was. I was to the point with myself that I kept telling myself I needed to somehow will all my problems into my really bad and painful right leg and then I'd have it cut off.

Soon after this time I talked to a good friend from my school days and told her what was going on with me. She said, "Why don't you go see my chiropractor". My reply was, "What are you going to a chiropractor for". She answered, "For the migraines I had". I knew nothing about chiropractic or chiropractors and asked "How will that help anything. I thought they were for back pain". She informed me of the thing I had not thought of during the conversation and that is NERVES and nerve pressure. What I didn't realize is that the bones and/or muscle can pinch nerves and you don't have to have spinal pain for it to happen. I hit the library again and made an appointment with the chiropractor she was seeing.

When I got to the chiropractor and had x-rays done, I was shocked with my spine. From the front –back view I had a 'S' shape. From the side view I had no natural bend in my spine at all. In fact my neck bowed almost totally backwards instead of having the frontal bend and my upper back bowed forward instead of backwards. I also had bones flung out right to left and also twisted right and left. This explained all of my leg and arm pain, strange heart spells I had when I tried to bend over and other really strange symptoms like raw, bleeding skin, crooked vision and a constant feeling like someone was pulling my feet and legs up within me as if I was being turned inside out. Also at 5 feet 8 inches I was only 105 pounds and I ate like a horse.

As I had been reading those library books, I knew we all have three nervous symptoms along with what each does. I asked really pointed questions as to what and where concerning what my x-rays showed and my strange problems and pains. I began treatments that day.

Six months later I could see improvement with myself. I knew it took about six months for one inch of nerve to heal or rejuvenate, so I was not giving up.

To add to the cure with myself, I found ONE listing in the phone book under 'Preventative Medicine' in the medical doctor area. I made a call and was there within the month. After various tests the insurance company didn't want to pay for, I was diagnosed with severe allergies to some things and some pretty heavy vitamin and mineral deficiencies. I was told my adrenals were exhausted, and that I didn't have enough zinc and iron in my body to stay alive. For the iron problem I was told to eat chicken livers every day because taking an iron supplement would only constipate me. Come to find out, the constant black spots shooting right and left that I always saw were gone within a couple of weeks after starting the liver snacks. I stayed on the chicken livers although I hate them. I was told the white spots all over my finger nails was due to the zinc I was missing. The preventative medicine doctor had me on all types of various vitamins and minerals three times a day. I was also taken off of all artificial ingredients and preservatives. The worst allergy I had was yeast and molds. That meant everything I stuck in my mouth I couldn't have it. It had to be 100% pure fresh food with no condiments and even a glass of pop or bottled juice was forbidden.

Little by little with all the extra nutrition I was taking, the food cleanout and the chiropractic treatments, I was coming back to normal. I couldn't figure out how my nutrition level was so bad as I was the colorful, fully balanced cook. I later learned that if the nutrients are not in the ground, it won't be in the foods and with meats it was the same story with what they ate. With the damage I had within me, I was also using up the nutrients fast.

As I found myself getting better I knew I had to start my son in with both of my newly found miracles. I made the appointments and he began first with the chiropractor. My son was really apprehensive with both appointments as he was really tired of being messed with and all the doctors.

His x-rays showed some major problems. I had to shake my head and I even commented to the chiropractor that the school spinal exams that they did hadn't picked up any problem. He had major problems with his neck, upper back, mid and lower back. X-rays were done of his spine by the chiropractor with and without the special shoes on. When I saw those x-rays the memory of the forceps and marks on the temples of my infant son was front and center. Now I realized that the doctor who delivered my son snapped the vertebra in his neck out of place and when he began to walk, it affected his entire spine with gravity and balance, hence tossing his spine totally out of place. That falls right in with my memory of how he seemed to decline when he began walking.

The preventive medicine doctor found major problems with him too. He was again diagnosed with severe allergies which we already knew and were getting allergy shots for. He was put on a total of ten things he could eat and drink and was told to be on that diet for three months. It was horrid for him as what he could have was things like tea, veal and the rest I do not remember. After that time frame we were to begin introducing a new food each week. I had a heck of a time trying to monitor what went into his mouth when I wasn't looking or around. He also had major vitamin and mineral deficiencies, some very different than mine. He was given strict orders of no artificial anything and no preservatives so I'd take him to the health food store to pick out kid stuff when he was allowed further foods.

We were both now taking bowls of vitamins and minerals three times a day with retesting done every few months and we were both under chiropractic care. My son was still following thru with all else as usual that we were dealing with for him but I never said a word to any of his doctors about what else I was doing.

It was very slow going but things began to improve with my son. One odd thing that happened was about two years after he began chiropractic care and it was right after he had a chiropractic appointment. He had an asthma attack seemingly from the spinal adjustment. The very next week on a usual Wednesday evening when we went to get his allergy shot, he then had a heavy duty asthma attack afterwards. He had received the shot and we headed home. When home about twenty minutes he began to wheeze, his throat began to close and he was into a really heavy attack. I quickly got the emergency pills for him that didn't really work well this time. That doctors office was closed by that time so the first thing the next morning I called the office and told them what had happened. The nurse said he had an attack from his shot and to bring him in that afternoon for an emergency retest.

We went back thru all the retesting and then went for the results appointment. At that time the nurse came in and said, "What have you been doing with this child. We've never seen anything like this. He's gone from the worst patient we had to having no allergies. If we don't get him off of the shots, the shots are going to kill him". I didn't answer her question right then as I let her set up his schedule to wean him off of the shots. After that I said, "To answer your question, I've been taking him to a chiropractor". Before I could say anything more, she looked at me, slowly walked backwards, left the room still walking backwards, then while still staring at me she walked sideways and was quickly gone down the hallway. I never talked to or saw her again. It took six or eight weeks as I remember to get him totally free of the shots. I still have to chuckle at that backwards walk. One thing was for sure and that was something within his body that was not working right was sure working now. I will always wonder if that attack he had the preceding week after the chiropractic appointment was actually the day his severe allergy woes ended and the attack was a reaction. His immune system was drastically changing for the better.

It was good news with the orthopedic surgeon too. The stunted leg began to grow and that doctor still monitored it every few months. It was really great when the redo on those shoes finally meant a smaller lift on the bottom of the shorter leg shoe. During the last visit there the doctor made a statement about the sudden rapid growth of the shorter leg. I made a statement saying, "I've been taking him to a chiropractor" and he didn't like that all, not one bit. He made it very clear that we were at the end of that appointment. I remember getting a call at some point where a nurse from there asked me if I wanted to schedule surgery to stop growth in the good leg. I told her no, not at this time. Her reply was that it had to be done by a certain age. My reply back was, "The short leg is growing. No surgery". We never went back to that office.

About those horrid school woes, they improved. He went from a first grade reader just into the early teens to a third grade reader quickly when things overall began to improve. The school system moved him up on the type of schooling he was getting as he was showing progress. He was no longer sitting in a room drawing all day long but he was with younger students which he did not like.

Chapter Four – The End Results

The end results with my son are really good. Now after at thirty years of independence from his mom, he still no longer has the allergy and asthma problems as he did have. Cut grass does bother him and he can't eat some preservative foods, although he should not eat any. An example for 'preservatives' is pizza he got by the register at a gas station that sells it as fresh baked pizza. Recently that pizza put him in the hospital twice for possible heart trouble. The second time made him realize what the problem was.

He can't read like a scholar, but he does pretty well. He is lost with big words but he is functional. A parent with a child having severe learning problems will understand this.

He ended up quitting school at age 19 as there was no way he could catchup to being in the senior class with others his age and he didn't like the stigma. He always has a job and goes to work every day. He has two grown children of his own now, one who just spent four years as a United States Marine.

His short leg never fully caught up and he should have a slight shoe lift which he won't do. He is a lot taller than he would have been had I given in for that 'destroy the growth node' surgery. Had the surgery been done he would now stand at about five feet, seven inches. Instead he now stands at almost six feet tall. It's a shame I didn't find out about chiropractic sooner.

As far as I know since my last conversation with him concerning his toilet woes, they are about nil or gone. That is a subject he just does not want to talk to me about. I think that problem was brought on from all the antibiotics the family doctor had him on when he was a small boy. I do keep mentioning to him to be sure and take probiotics.

With me, I became the shopper at the grocery that reads all the labels. I know what many of the ingredient terms mean and how things can have hidden meanings. One thing I warn people about is monosodium glutamate. Its history began many, many centuries ago being putrefied fish heads in clay pots that was added to foods. Now it can be found under the term of 'natural'. An example of what it did to a member of my family is my father. It took some experiments to figure out why at times he would lose his upper vision. It was always within twenty-four hours after eating MSG.

As far as my strange medical woes, I'm doing really great. I do have nerve damage, like not having full feeling in a leg, but I deal with it and no one notices.

The old saying of 'you are what you eat' is definitely true. I know there are no magic monsters running around in the body. I have come to the conclusion that if it is contagious it is a disease. Otherwise when something is wrong, not working correctly, it is a disorder.

Now I also do understand how nutrition can affect anything within the body as does spinal problems, that including how the nutrition needs by each specific person can be very different in different ways.

I keep reminding my son that he has to have his spine maintained a few times each year and at times I mention that he cannot survive on a diet of junk and crappy foods. At this point he is responsible for himself but as with most moms, I'm still hovering and get 'that look' for doing so!